LUPUS

DIET COOKBOOK

DELICIOUS AND EASY ANTI INFLAMMATORY RECIPES TO LIVE HEALTHY AND MANAGE LUPUS

Mildred A. Kelly

SCAN QR CODE BELOW TO GAIN ACCESS TO MORE BOOKS BY THE AUTHOR

About The Author Page

Mildred A Kelly is a passionate chef who focuses on healthy eating and lifestyle. She creates wholesome, delicious, and health-conscious meals that are both tasty and accessible.

With a background in fresh, wholesome foods, Mildred believes that the path to healthier living begins in the kitchen. She is the creator of several exceptional cookbooks, each a testament to her passion for promoting well-being through tasty, thoughtfully created meals.

Her recipes are a blend of culinary expertise and a true awareness of nutritional demands. These cookbooks are not just compilations of recipes; they are invitations to start a journey of flavor, health, and joy in the kitchen.

Mildred's recipes are a testament to her dedication to creating wonderful moments and a lifetime appreciation for the junction of taste and well-being.

TABLE OF CONTENTS

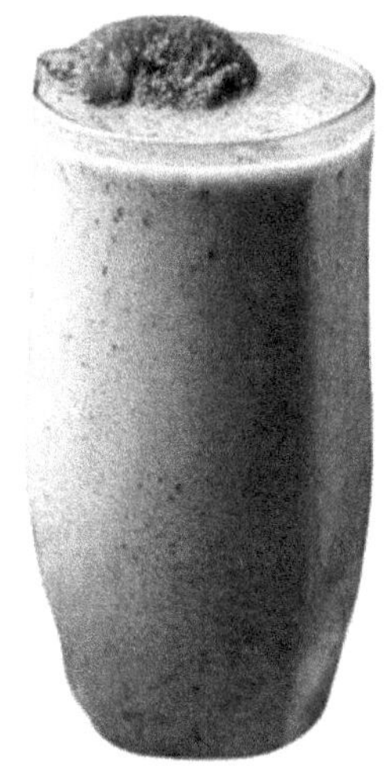

TROPICAL DETOX DELIGHT

Introduction

My heart was pounding in time with the rain pattering against the kitchen window. I gazed at the vacant plate I held, its stark whiteness belying the harmonious blend of tastes resonating in my mind. The colorful meal of Thai curry and roasted vegetables that was supposed to be served tonight was wilting in the compost bin due to another flare-up of lupus. Once a temple of taste discovery, my body felt now like a delicate melody that could quickly go out of tune.

I realized then that I needed to adjust the song. Not by muting the sound of pleasure, but by creating a brand-new symphony in which wellbeing and flavor are harmoniously blended. That resolve gave rise to this cookbook, which is proof that a lupus diet doesn't have to consist of boring dishes like steamed vegetables and boiled chicken. It can be a stirring salsa of hues, a heartfelt concerto of textures, or a colorful opera, all the while nourishing your body and aiding in the control of flare-ups.

Having spent years researching diets, I can attest to the transformational impact of a well-planned lupus diet. However, I've also witnessed the anguish, perplexity, and anxiety of forgoing flavor in favor of health. This book will serve as both your culinary compass and my bridge as it leads you through a world of mouthwatering and healthful options.

There's more in these pages than just recipes. A mindful eating philosophy, tactics for portion control for maximum health and flare management (with an extra bonus chapter!), and advice on turning every meal into a celebration of flavor and wellbeing are all included.

You'll become proficient at:

Accept attentive portion control: Learn how smaller, more balanced meals can improve digestion, lower inflammation, and aid with weight management.

Cook with confidence: Learn useful techniques for navigating supermarket aisles, understanding food labels, and preparing wholesome, filling meals in your own kitchen.

Taste the symphony of flavors: Discover a world of colorful meals that are brimming with nutrients, anti-inflammatory Ingredients, and sheer gastronomic bliss.

Satisfy your body, calm your mind: Acknowledge your hunger signals, honor your body's guidance, and relish the process of crafting a customized Lupus Diet plan.

This is more than simply a cookbook—it's a call to rediscover the bliss of eating, the beat of your own nutritional requirements, and the melodic harmony of wellbeing that emerges with every thoughtful mouthful. So, turn the page, grab your apron, and get ready to lead your own symphony of flavor and wellness. The tunes are ready.

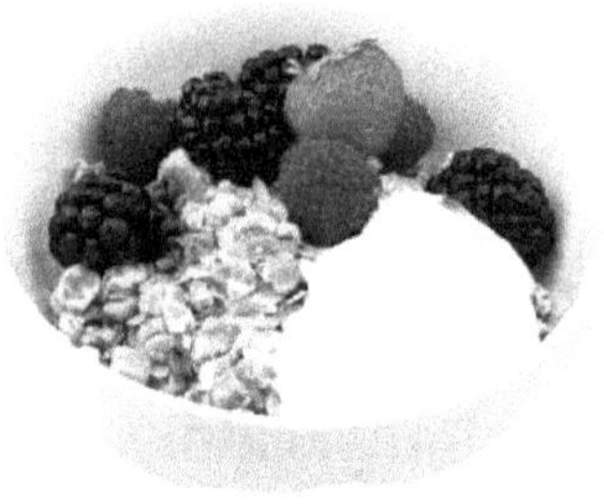

BERRY DELIGHT OATMEAL BOWL

Chapter 1: Getting Around with Lupus

Receiving a lupus diagnosis might be like entering a maze of unknowns. It can be quite daunting due to the disease's complexity, unpredictability, and effects on all facets of life. But among all of this turmoil, there is also room for composure, empathy, and proactive measures that will lead to a journey of greater empowerment and nourishment.

We'll examine the complex relationship between diet and lupus and how making thoughtful food choices can help manage symptoms and enhance general health.

Recognizing The Intricacies Of Lupus, Its Symptoms, And How It Affects Digestion

Systemic lupus erythematosus, sometimes known as lupus, is a chronic autoimmune illness in which healthy tissue is mistakenly attacked by the immune system, causing inflammation and damage to many parts of the body. Although anybody can be impacted by this complex and unpredictable disease, women and people of color are more likely to get it.

Getting Around the Maze of Symptoms:
As different as snowflakes, lupus symptoms can vary widely from person to person and even change over time.

The following are typical indications and symptoms:

Fatigue: An excessive and enduring state of exhaustion that interferes with day-to-day activity. Any joint might experience joint pain and swelling, which frequently occurs symmetrically and results in stiffness and discomfort.

Skin rashes: The characteristic "butterfly rash" over the cheeks and bridge of the nose, along with other photosensitive rashes.

Fever: Unexplained fever, often low-grade, that comes and goes.

Hair loss: Medication side effects or inflammation can cause diffuse or uneven hair loss.

Mouth sores: The inside of the mouth or tongue may become infected with painful ulcers.

Breathlessness and chest pain: These symptoms may be brought on by lung or pleural inflammation (inflammation of the lung lining). Certain cases may have neurological involvement, resulting in headaches, disorientation, and seizures.

Raynaud's phenomenon: Insufficient blood flow causing fingers and toes to turn white or blue.

Digestive Disarray and Lupus:

Lupus typically affects the digestive system, resulting in a variety of unpleasant symptoms that can seriously impair quality of life. These may consist of:

Vomiting and nausea: Usually brought on by gut or stomach irritation Increased stomach acid production can irritate the oesophagus, causing heartburn and acid reflux.

Pain and cramping in the abdomen: An irritated or inflamed digestive tract may result in discomfort. Constipation or diarrhea can cause erratic or unpredictable bowel motions.

Changes in appetite or loss of appetite: Cravings for strange foods or a lack of appetite are possible.

Swallowing difficulties: In extreme situations, inflammation may damage the oesophagus.

The Intertwined Threads:

The following elements contribute to the complexity of lupus and its effects on digestion:

Autoimmune attack: The digestive system's tissues may be attacked by the immune system, causing inflammation and damage.

Medication: Nausea, vomiting, or diarrhea are some of the side effects of some lupus drugs.

Anxiety and stress: These frequent companions of long-term sickness can exacerbate symptoms related to the stomach.

Nutritional deficiencies: Digestion-related malabsorption of nutrients might worsen general health.

Discovering the Way Through the Maze:
Although there is no known cure for lupus, it is feasible to manage its symptoms and lessen the

damage it does to your digestive system. The following are some crucial actions:

Collaborate with your physician: Keeping an eye on symptoms and modifying treatment strategies require frequent examinations and honest dialogue.
Adopt a nutritious diet: Pay special attention to anti-inflammatory foods such as whole grains, fruits, vegetables, and healthy fats. Control your stress by using calming methods like yoga, meditation, or deep breathing.
Remain hydrated: Eating enough water is crucial for healthy digestion and general wellbeing. Pay attention to what causes your stomach troubles and steer clear of such things in order to listen to your body.
Join a group for support: Making connections with people who are aware of your path might be really beneficial.

How Nutrition Can Help Control Lupus
It's a daily dance to manage the unexpected nature of lupus and figure out how to feel your best when you have it. Out of all of these, one sticks out as an effective tool: your nutrition. Not only fuel, the

foods you eat can have a big impact on your inflammation levels, lupus symptoms, and general health.

The Symphony of Anti-Inflammation:

The main feature of lupus is inflammation, which is a process that can seriously damage your body. A balanced diet can act as a conductor in this situation, arranging an anti-inflammatory symphony.

Fruits and vegetables are nature's superfoods for reducing inflammation! Berries (particularly blueberries, strawberries, and raspberries) abound in antioxidants that attack free radicals and reduce inflammation. Broccoli, tomatoes, bell peppers, and leafy greens are full of vitamins, minerals, and phytonutrients that slow down the processes that cause inflammation. To get the advantages of different antioxidants, try to arrange your food in a rainbow pattern.

Whole Grains: Choose whole grains such as brown rice, quinoa, and whole-wheat bread instead of processed carbohydrates. Because of their high fiber content, these complex carbohydrates control blood sugar, give long-lasting energy, and have anti-inflammatory properties. Additionally, fiber supports your gut microbiota, which is important for general health and may have an impact on lupus activity.

Good Fats: Rich in omega-3 fatty acids, fatty fish such as mackerel, salmon, and tuna have strong anti-inflammatory qualities. Nuts, seeds, avocados, and olive oil all provide vitamin E and good fats that help reduce inflammation.

Never undervalue the flavor-exploding power of spices and herbs! There are anti-inflammatory Ingredients in cayenne pepper, ginger, garlic, and turmeric that can help. Try including these to enhance the flavor and reduce inflammation in your meals.

Keeping Away from the Inflammatory Noise:

Certain foods may function as off-key instruments in your anti-inflammatory orchestra, while others may have a supporting role.

Processed Foods: Avoid processed foods because they are high in artificial Ingredients, refined sugars, and saturated and harmful fats. These may intensify lupus symptoms and cause inflammation.

Red Meat and Processed Meats: Steer clear of processed meats, such as bacon and sausages. These may raise the chance of flare-ups and lead to inflammation.

Dairy: For some lupus sufferers, dairy products exacerbate their symptoms. Observe your reaction to dairy and modify your intake accordingly.

Gluten: Although not all lupus patients have a sensitivity to gluten, some report that being gluten-free helps their symptoms. Try other things to determine whether gluten is a trigger for you.

Sugar: Consuming too much sugar can damage gut health and exacerbate inflammation. Reduce your intake of sweets, processed carbs, and sugary drinks to manage your inflammation.

Finding Your Food Triggers by Silencing the Noise

As distinct as every individual's experience with lupus, dietary sensitivity might differ significantly. Finding your unique triggers requires some research, but the benefits are substantial.

Record Your Meals and Symptoms for a Few Weeks Using a Food Diary. Look for trends: does a particular food usually come on before a flare-up or an increase in symptoms?

Elimination Diet: For information on implementing an elimination diet, speak with a medical practitioner or qualified dietitian. This entails eliminating possible trigger foods for a predetermined amount of time, then progressively reintroducing them to see how your body reacts.

Testing for food sensitivity: Certain tests can reveal possible food sensitivities, even though they are not always definitive. While using this material as a reference, remember to always put in the order of personal observation and medical advice.

Recall that following a healthy diet is a journey rather than a destination. Try new meals, research them, and give them priority when it comes to how you feel. Accept the instruments of a well-balanced diet to perform your own internal anti-inflammatory symphony, which will assist you in managing and overcoming lupus.

Chapter 2: Anti-inflammatory Powerhouse Ingredients

Visualize your kitchen as a lively marketplace filled with nutrient-rich Ingredients, appealing fragrances, and brilliant colors that will feed your wellness and fight off the inflammatory forces linked to lupus. We'll look at the superfoods that are low in inflammation in this chapter—fruits, vegetables, whole grains, and healthy fats—so that you may make wise decisions for your lupus journey.

Fruits & Vegetables: A Symphony

The abundance of nature provides a range of anti-inflammatory heroes, each contributing a different note to your inner harmony of health.

Berries: Packed full of antioxidants, especially the powerful anti-inflammatory anthocyanins found in them, berries are small jewels. Strawberries, raspberries, cherries, and blueberries are a few examples of berries that can help lower inflammation, shield cells from harm, and even enhance cognitive performance.

Leafy Greens: Savor the health benefits of arugula, collard greens, spinach, and kale. These vegetables are bursting with vitamins, minerals, and phytonutrients like sulforaphane, which may reduce inflammation and even stave against chronic illnesses. Never undervalue the humble lettuce: butter and romaine are rich in folate, which is essential for the health and repair of cells.

Bell peppers: These colorful jewels are excellent sources of vitamin C, an antioxidant that boosts immunity and reduces inflammation. Another powerful anti-inflammatory substance, lycopene, is especially abundant in red bell peppers. Go beyond the traditional red pepper and try the diversity of nutrients and flavors that orange, yellow, and green peppers offer.

Broccoli and Cruciferous Cousins: The cruciferous family, which includes cabbage, cauliflower, Brussels sprouts, and broccoli, is well-known for its glucosinolates, which decompose into substances that reduce inflammation. In addition, these veggies are a great source of vitamins and fiber, which support intestinal health and wellbeing in general.

Whole Grains: The Nutritional Heartbeat:

Give up processed carbohydrates and enjoy the long-lasting energy and anti-inflammatory properties of whole grains.

Quinoa: Packed with fiber, magnesium, and manganese, this ancient grain rich in protein is free of gluten and can help lower inflammation while promoting general health.

Grains of Brown Rice: Brown rice is a flexible and high-fiber substitute for white rice that helps control blood sugar levels and offers long-lasting energy. To add even more antioxidants and a nutty flavor, try wild rice.

Whole-Wheat Pastas and Bread: Steer clear of refined grains and choose whole-wheat alternatives.

For optimal benefits in terms of fiber and nutrients, look for breads and pastas that have at least 80% whole wheat.

Healthy Fats: The Melody of Lubrication

Don't be afraid of fats; the correct kind can calm your inflammatory pathways like a gentle song.

Omega-3 Fatty Acids: Superstars at lowering inflammation, omega-3s can be found in fatty fish like salmon, tuna, mackerel, and sardines. To get the benefits of its preventive qualities, try to eat two servings of fatty fish every week.

Olive Oil: An essential component of the Mediterranean diet, olive oil is high in antioxidants and monounsaturated fats, such as oleocanthal, which has anti-inflammatory properties. Use it for mild cooking or to drizzle over salads and vegetables.

Avocados: Packed with heart-healthy monounsaturated fats, fiber, potassium, and vitamin E, these creamy treats also help reduce inflammation and promote heart health. Savor them with a squeeze of lemon and a pinch of salt, or just mashed and added to salads and sandwiches.

Nuts and Seeds: Rich in fiber, good fats, and minerals like zinc and magnesium, almonds, walnuts, chia seeds, flaxseeds, and hemp seeds all help to control inflammation. You can eat them as a nutritious snack or sprinkle them over salads and yogurt.

The Magic of Spice: Balancing Your Recipes

Never undervalue the ability of herbs and spices to flavor food and provide anti-inflammatory benefits.

Turmeric: Packed with of health benefits, curcumin is a powerful anti-inflammatory component found in this golden spice. It can be added to smoothies, soups, curries, and even golden milk for a tasty and healing boost.

Ginger: Known for its pain-relieving and anti-inflammatory qualities, gingerols are present in this warming spice. Savor it with teas, stir-fries, or even grated in meat and vegetable marinades.

Garlic and onions: These flavorful mainstays have anti-inflammatory qualities due to their contents of quercetin and allicin, respectively.

Recipe Substitutions for Combustible Substances

Now that you are aware of which fruits, veggies, whole grains, and healthy fats are the best anti-inflammatory foods, let's make use of them! Changing out inflammatory foods with tasty and nutritious substitutes can make a big difference in your lupus journey. Here are a few motivational swaps:

Give Up Saturated Fat:

- **Instead Of:** Fried meals, creamy sauces, and fatty meat portions
- **Try:** Vegetable broth-based sauces, baked tofu, salmon, poultry breast, and lentil pasta are examples of lean protein sources.

Get Rid of Refined Carbs:

- **Instead Of:** Sugary cereals, white bread, spaghetti, and pastries
- **Try:** Quinoa, brown rice, oats, fruit and nut combinations, whole-wheat bread and pasta.

Cut Down on Added Sugar:

- **Swap:** Sugary Drinks like sodas, Candy, and Sugar-Rich Desserts
- **Try:** Smoothies made with unsweetened almond milk, fresh or frozen fruits, and baked products created from scratch that are naturally sweetened with honey or maple syrup.

Avoid gluten if necessary:

- **In place of:** Rye, barley, and wheat flour
- **Try:** buckwheat flour, quinoa flour, almond flour, coconut flour, and gluten-free pasta and bread choices.

Spice Things Up:

- **Instead of:** blad foods that lack an anti-inflammatory punch, add some spiciness to your life.
- **Try:** cloves, cinnamon, rosemary, cayenne pepper, ginger, garlic, onions, and turmeric.

Inspiration for a Recipe:

To help you get started, try these particular recipe substitutions:

- **Replace creamy chicken Alfredo**: with baked salmon seasoned with herbs and roasted veggies.
- **Replace your Sugary Breakfast cereal:** with overnight oats flavored with chia seeds and berries.
- **Forego the fried chicken wings in favor of:** Air-fried tofu bites with a spicy dipping sauce
- **Put down the white bread toast and turn toward:** Avocado toast made with whole wheat and feta cheese crumbles

Although powerful anti-inflammatory Ingredients are essential for lupus management, keep in mind that health is a whole symphony. To live your best life with lupus, incorporate a nutritious diet, frequent exercise, restful sleep, stress-reduction strategies, and building relationships with your support network.

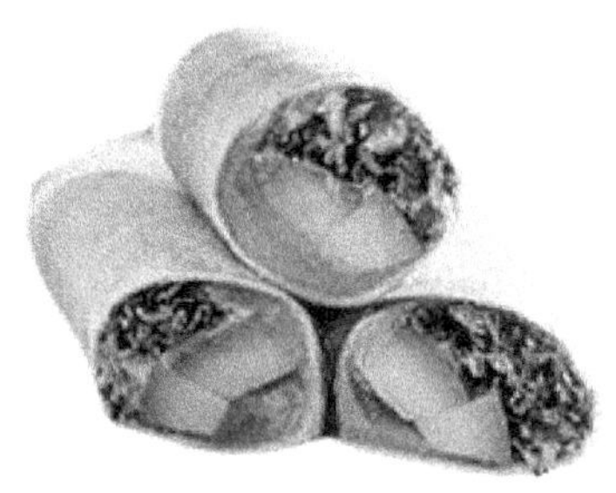

SMOKED SALMON AND AVOCADO WRAPS WITH SPROUTS

Chapter 3: Building Your Lupus Pantry: Essential staples for a Lupus-friendly kitchen

Think of your kitchen as a health-conscious oasis, full with colorful elements that are just waiting to play a harmonious, anti-inflammatory tune inside your body. We'll cover the fundamentals of creating a lupus-friendly pantry in this chapter, giving you the information and techniques to shop wisely, feel confident in the supermarket aisles, and cook meals to optimize their nutritional value.

The Crucial Group:

The main Ingredients in your lupus-friendly pantry are as follows:

Vegetables and Fruits: Fill up on a spectrum of hues! Your best allies against inflammation are berries (strawberries, raspberries, blueberries), leafy greens (kale, collard greens, spinach), bell peppers (orange, red, yellow), broccoli, and cruciferous veggies (brussels sprouts, cauliflower). For year-round availability and convenience, don't overlook frozen options.

Complete Grains: Give up processed carbohydrates and embrace the fiber and long-lasting energy of whole grains. Quinoa, brown rice, whole-wheat bread and pasta, and gluten-free alternatives like buckwheat and millet offer numerous options.

Healthy Fats: Omega-3-rich fatty seafood (salmon, tuna, mackerel, sardines) is important. Plant-based omega-3 fatty acids and monounsaturated fats can be found in avocados, olive oil, almonds, walnuts, chia, flax, and hemp seeds.

Spices and Herbs: Flavor and anti-inflammatory properties are added by turmeric, ginger, garlic, onions, cayenne pepper, cinnamon, rosemary, and cloves.

Protein Sources: Fish, tofu, skinless chicken breast, and legumes (beans, lentils) are excellent sources of lean protein that are essential for both gaining and preserving muscle mass.

Dairy substitutes: For people who cannot consume dairy, unsweetened nut milks made from almond, cashew, or coconut as well as plant-based yogurts provide calcium and vitamin D.

How to Handle the Grocery Symphony

- **Pay close attention to the labels:** Pay attention to whole foods and stay away from processed foods that are high in sodium, saturated fats, and added sugars.
- **Seek out credentials:** To reduce your exposure to pesticides, whenever possible, use organic produce. Dairy and meat from grass-fed cattle have more nutrients.
- **Make a meal plan:** Make a grocery list that is based on your meal plan in order to prevent impulsive buys and food waste.
- **Remember to consider canned and frozen foods:** Convenience and fiber are provided by canned beans, while frozen fruits and vegetables can be just as nutrient-dense as fresh ones.

Proper Food Storage

Proper food storage and preparation preserves nutrients and reduces factors that cause inflammation:

- Thoroughly wash fruits and vegetables.
- Fruits and vegetables should be kept in the refrigerator's crisper drawer.
- To save cooking leftovers again, split them out and freeze them.
- Make use of cooking techniques like grilling, baking, steaming, or stir-frying that help retain nutrients.
- Avoid deep-frying and excessive oil use.
- For beans to have less potentially inflammatory lectins, soak and boil them properly.

Past the Pantry Walls

Keep in mind that your lupus-friendly pantry is only one piece in the whole orchestra of your health. To create a holistic symphony of empowerment and sustenance on your lupus journey, incorporate mindful grocery shopping, food storage, and preparation practices with other healthful habits like exercise, stress management, and sleep management.

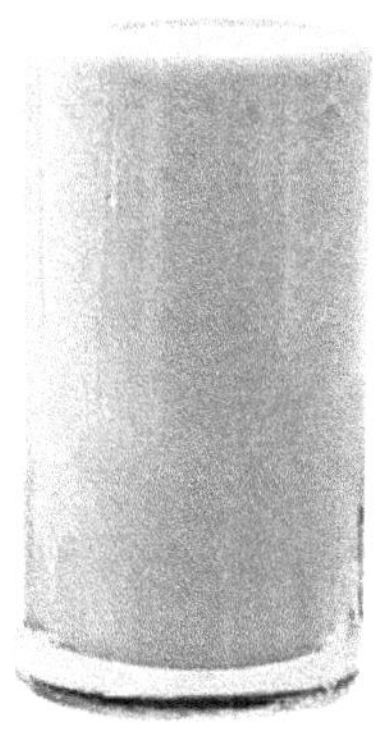

TROPICAL POWER SMOOTHIE

Berry Delight Oatmeal Bowl (Gluten-Free & Vegan)

- **Prep Time:** 5 minutes
- **Serves:** 1

Ingredients

- Half a cup of rolled oats (if necessary, certified gluten-free)
- 1 cup almond milk without sugar
- 1/4 cup of frozen or fresh mixed berries
- One spoonful of chia seeds
- half a teaspoon of cinnamon powder
- 1/4 cup of walnuts, chopped (optional)

Instructions

- In a saucepan, mix together oats, almond milk, cinnamon, and chia seeds. After bringing to a boil, simmer for five minutes while stirring now and then.

- Turn off the heat and allow to cool a little.
- Add berries and, if desired, walnuts on top.
- Have fun!

Nutritional Value:
- Calories: 300
- Fiber: 10 grams
- Protein: 8 grams
- Fat: 10 grams (healthy fats from chia seeds and walnuts)
- Antioxidants: Rich in berries and spices

Turmeric Scramble with Spinach and Avocado

- **Prep Time:** 10 minutes
- **Serves:** 1

Ingredients
- two eggs
- 1/4 cup of finely chopped spinach
- 1/4 of an avocado, cut up
- 1/4 tsp powdered turmeric
- A dash of dark pepper

- One tablespoon of olive oil

Instructions

- In a pan over medium heat, warm the olive oil.
- Beat eggs with pepper and turmeric.
- Transfer the egg mixture to the pan and cook it completely by scrambling it.
- Add the spinach and cook for a further one minute.
- Garnish with sliced avocado and serve with whole-wheat toast, if desired.

Nutritional Value:

- Calories: 350
- Fiber: 3 grams
- Protein: 15 grams
- Fat: 20 grams (healthy fats from avocado and olive oil)
- Anti-inflammatory benefits: Turmeric and spinach

Chia Seed Pudding with Berries and Nuts

- **Prep Time:** 10 minutes (plus overnight soaking)
- **Serves:** 1

Ingredients

- One-fourth cup of chia seeds
- 1 cup almond milk without sugar
- 1/4 cup of frozen or fresh mixed berries
- One tablespoon of chopped nuts, such as pecans, walnuts, or almonds
- 1/4 tsp (optional) vanilla extract
- Taste-tested honey or maple syrup (optional)

Instructions

- In a jar or bowl, mix the chia seeds, almond milk, and vanilla extract (if using). Give it a good stir, then refrigerate for the entire night.
- Add nuts and berries on top in the morning. If desired, drizzle with maple syrup or honey.

Nutritional Value:

- Calories: 250
- Fiber: 10 grams
- Protein: 5 grams
- Fat: 15 grams (healthy fats from chia seeds and nuts)
- Omega-3 fatty acids: Chia seeds

Tropical Power Smoothie

- **Prep Time:** 5 minutes
- **Serves:** 1

Ingredients

- 1 cup coconut milk without sugar
- half of a frozen banana
- one-fourth cup frozen mango
- 1/4 cup frozen or fresh pineapple chunks
- one-fourth cup spinach
- One spoonful of chia seeds
- Half a teaspoon of optional ginger powder

Instructions

- Fill a blender with all the ingredients; process until smooth.
- Have fun!

Nutritional Value:

- Calories: 300
- Fiber: 5 grams
- Protein: 5 grams
- Fat: 10 grams (healthy fats from coconut milk)
- Vitamins and minerals: Packed with fruits and vegetables

Savory Protein Frittata with Sweet Potato and Greens

- **Prep Time:** 15 minutes
- **Serves:** 2

Ingredients

- 4 eggs
- 1/2 cup chopped spinach or kale, and 1/2 cup diced sweet potatoes

- 1/4 cup of finely chopped red onion
- 1/4 cup of feta cheese, crumbled
- One tsp olive oil
- To taste, add salt and pepper.

Instructions
- Set oven temperature to 200°C/400°F.
- In an oven-safe pan or cast-iron skillet, warm the olive oil over medium heat. Cook the chopped sweet potato for five to seven minutes, or until it becomes tender.
- Cook the chopped onion for a further two to three minutes, or until it becomes tender.
- Add the spinach or kale and simmer for an additional minute, or until it wilts.
- In a bowl, whisk together the eggs, pepper, and salt.
- Add the egg mixture to the pan with the veggies and gently whisk to blend.
- Top with feta cheese that has been crushed.
- Place the pan in the oven and bake for fifteen to twenty minutes, or until the top is browned and the eggs are set.

- Before slicing and serving, allow it cool slightly.

Nutritional Value:
- Calories: 250 per serving
- Fiber: 2 grams per serving
- Protein: 15 grams per serving
- Fat: 10 grams per serving (healthy fats from olive oil and feta cheese)
- Antioxidants: Rich in sweet potato and greens

Tips:
- Feel free to add more veggies if you'd like, such bell peppers, mushrooms, or zucchini.
- Try using a different kind of cheese, like mozzarella or goat cheese.
- Accompany the frittata with avocado slices or whole-wheat bread.

Mediterranean Quinoa Salad with Grilled Chicken and Lemon Dill Dressing

- **Prep Time:** 20 minutes (plus grilling time)
- **Serves:** 1-2

Ingredients

- 1 cup of quinoa, cooked
- half a grilled, sliced chicken breast
- half a cup of cucumber, chopped
- half a cup of chopped tomatoes
- 1/4 cup of coarsely chopped red onion
- Half a cup of Kalamata olives
- 1/4 cup of feta cheese, crumbled
- One tablespoon of olive oil
- One tablespoon of lemon juice
- Half a teaspoon of dried dill
- To taste, add salt and pepper.

Instructions

- Slice and grill the chicken breast.
- 2. Transfer the quinoa, chicken, red onion, cucumber, tomato, olives, and feta cheese into a bowl.
- 3. In a small bowl, whisk together olive oil, lemon juice, dill, salt, and pepper. After pouring, toss to coat the salad.
- 4. Have fun!

Nutritional Value:

- Calories: 400
- Fiber: 6 grams
- Protein: 30 grams
- Fat: 15 grams (healthy fats from olives and olive oil)
- Anti-inflammatory benefits: Tomatoes, olive oil, and spices

Smoked Salmon and Avocado Wraps with Sprouts

- **Prep Time:** 10 minutes
- **Serves:** 1-2

Ingredients

- Two tacos made using whole wheat
- Two tablespoons of cream cheese (dairy-free or low-fat)
- Two pieces of smoked salmon
- Half an avocado, cut into slices
- 1/4 cup of sprouting alfalfa
- Sprigs of dill (optional)

Instructions

- Top each tortilla with a layer of cream cheese.
- Add sprouts, avocado slices, and smoked salmon on top.
- Roll up tortillas; if preferred, fasten with toothpicks.
- Garnish with dill sprigs (optional).

Nutritional Value:

- Calories: 350
- Fiber: 4 grams
- Protein: 20 grams

- Fat: 15 grams (healthy fats from avocado and salmon)
- Omega-3 fatty acids: Smoked salmon

Lentil Soup with Whole-Wheat Bread and Herbs

- **Prep Time:** 30 minutes
- **Serves:** 4

Ingredients
- 1 cup washed green lentils
- 1 cup of sliced carrots and 4 cups of vegetable broth
- one cup of celery, chopped
- 1/2 cup finely chopped onion; 2 minced garlic cloves
- A single tsp of dried thyme
- Half a teaspoon of rosemary, dried
- To taste, add salt and pepper.
- Sliced whole-wheat bread
- Garnish with fresh herbs (parsley, cilantro, etc.)

Instructions

- Fill a saucepan with lentils, stock, celery, onion, garlic, thyme, and rosemary. Once the lentils are cooked, simmer for 20 to 25 minutes on low heat after bringing to a boil.
- 2. To taste, add salt and pepper for seasoning.
- 3. Garnish the soup with fresh herbs and serve it with slices of whole-wheat bread.

Nutritional Value:

- Calories: 250 per serving
- Fiber: 5 grams per serving
- Protein: 15 grams per serving
- Iron and folate: Rich in lentils
- Antioxidants: From vegetables and herbs

Thai Vegetable Curry with Brown Rice

- **Prep Time:** 20 minutes
- **Serves:** 2

Ingredients

- 1 tsp olive oil

- One sliced red bell pepper
- One sliced green bell pepper
- one cup florets of broccoli
- half a cup of finely sliced zucchini
- 1/4 cup finely chopped onion and 2 minced garlic cloves
- One can (13.5 oz) milk from coconuts
- One spoonful of paste made from red curry.
- One spoonful of soy sauce
- Half a teaspoon of powdered ginger
- 1/4 cup of freshly chopped cilantro
- One cup of brown rice, cooked

Instructions

- In a pan over medium heat, warm the olive oil. Add onion, bell peppers, broccoli, and zucchini. Cook, stirring periodically, for 5 to 7 minutes.
- Cook the garlic for one additional minute.
- Add the ginger powder, soy sauce, coconut milk, and red curry paste. After bringing to a simmer, cook the vegetables for five minutes, or until they are soft.

- Serve cooked brown rice with a stir-in of chopped cilantro.

Nutritional Value:
- Calories: 400
- Fiber: 8 grams
- Protein: 10 grams
- Fat: 15 grams (healthy fats from coconut milk)
- Anti-inflammatory benefits: Curry spices, turmeric in curry paste, vegetables

Turkey and Veggie Salad with Whole-Wheat Pita Bread

- **Prep Time:** 15 minutes
- **Serves:** 1-2

Ingredients
- 1 toasted whole-wheat pita bread
- 3 ounces grilled or roasted, sliced lean turkey breast
- half a cup of baby spinach
- 1/4 cup of cucumbers, chopped

- 1/4 cup of finely chopped red onion
- one-fourth cup finely chopped tomatoes
- One tablespoon of hummus
- One tablespoon of lemon juice
- One-half tsp dried oregano
- To taste, add salt and pepper.

Instructions

- Top the hot pita bread with hummus.
- Add spinach, turkey, cucumber, tomato, and red onion on top.
- In a small bowl, whisk together lemon juice, oregano, salt, and pepper. Pour over the greens.
- Have fun!

Nutritional Value:

- Calories: 350
- Fiber: 5 grams
- Protein: 25 grams
- Fat: 10 grams (healthy fats from hummus)
- Vitamin C and potassium: Rich in vegetables

Extra Tips:

- Feel free to alter these recipes to suit your dietary requirements and preferences.
- Use your imagination when preparing leftovers! You can load bell peppers with leftover quinoa salad, turn leftover curry into a filling lentil bowl, and eat leftovers with salad greens.
- When you're on the go, you can still enjoy a satisfying and tasty meal by packing your lunch in an insulated container to keep it fresh.

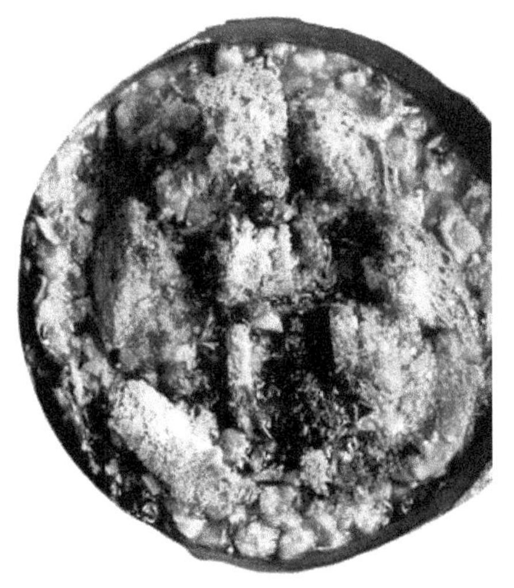

LENTIL SOUP WITH WHOLE-WHEAT BREAD AND HERBS

Chapter 6: Dinner Recipes

Salmon with Roasted Vegetables and Lemon Dill Sauce

- **Prep Time:** 20 minutes (plus grilling time)
- **Serves:** 2

Ingredients

- 2 fillets of salmon
- One tablespoon of olive oil
- To taste, add salt and pepper.
- Chopped broccoli florets, one cup
- one cup of finely chopped asparagus
- half a cup of cherry tomatoes
- 1/4 cup finely sliced red onion
- One tablespoon of lemon juice
- Half a teaspoon of dried dill
- 1/4 cup low-fat or lactose-free plain Greek yogurt

Instructions

- Set oven temperature to 200°C/400°F.

- Use salt, pepper, and olive oil to season the salmon fillets.
- Combine olive oil, salt, and pepper with broccoli, asparagus, tomatoes, and red onion. Place on an oven tray and cook for 15 to 20 minutes, or until soft.
- In the interim, cook the salmon fillets through by grilling or pan-frying them.
- Combine Greek yogurt, dill, and lemon juice in a small bowl.
- Place the salmon fillet on a plate, cover with roasted veggies, and pour lemon-dill sauce over it.

Nutritional Value:
- Calories: 450
- Fiber: 5 grams
- Protein: 35 grams
- Fat: 20 grams (healthy fats from salmon and olive oil)
- Omega-3 fatty acids: Salmon
- Anti-inflammatory benefits: Dill, vegetables

Mediterranean Chickpea and Vegetable Bowl with Whole-Wheat Couscous

- **Prep Time:** 15 minutes
- **Serves:** 2

Ingredients

- 1 cup cooked couscous made with whole wheat
- One can (15 oz) of rinsed and drained chickpeas
- half a cup of cucumber, chopped
- half a cup of chopped tomatoes
- 1/4 cup of feta cheese, crumbled
- Half a cup of Kalamata olives
- 1/4 cup of coarsely chopped red onion
- One tablespoon of olive oil
- One tablespoon of lemon juice
- One-half tsp dried oregano
- To taste, add salt and pepper.

Instructions

- Use a fork to fluff the cooked couscous.

- Combine couscous, chickpeas, cucumber, tomato, feta cheese, olives, and red onion in a bowl.
- In a small bowl, whisk together olive oil, lemon juice, oregano, salt, and pepper. Over the salad, drizzle, then toss to coat.

Nutritional Value:
- Calories: 400
- Fiber: 7 grams
- Protein: 20 grams
- Fat: 15 grams (healthy fats from olives and olive oil)
- Iron and protein: Rich in chickpeas
- Antioxidants: From vegetables and spices

Thai Coconut Curry with Tofu and Brown Rice

- **Prep Time:** 20 minutes
- **Serves:** 2

Ingredients
- 1 tsp olive oil

- One sliced red bell pepper, one sliced green bell pepper, one can (13.5 oz) of cubed and pan-fried tofu milk from coconuts
- One spoonful of paste made from red curry.
- One spoonful of soy sauce
- Half a teaspoon of powdered ginger
- one cup of freshly chopped spinach
- One cup of brown rice, cooked

Instructions

- In a pan over medium heat, warm the olive oil. Cook the tofu until it turns golden brown on all sides.
- Add the bell peppers and simmer, stirring periodically, for 5 minutes.
- Add the ginger powder, soy sauce, coconut milk, and red curry paste. After bringing to a simmer, cook the vegetables for five minutes, or until they are soft.
- Add the spinach and stir-fry it until it wilts.
- Top cooked brown rice with curry.

Nutritional Value:

- Calories: 450

- Fiber: 5 grams
- Protein: 25 grams
- Fat: 15 grams (healthy fats from coconut milk)
- Anti-inflammatory benefits: Curry spices, turmeric in curry paste

Creamy Lemon Chicken with Broccoli and Quinoa

- **Prep Time:** 20 minutes
- **Serves:** 2

Ingredients
- 2 chicken breasts, skinless and boneless
- One tablespoon of olive oil
- To taste, add salt and pepper
- 1/2 cup finely chopped onion
- 2 minced garlic cloves
- One cup of chicken broth and half a cup of low-fat Greek yogurt
- one-fourth cup lemon juice
- 1/4 tsp powdered turmeric
- One cup of cooked quinoa

* one cup florets of broccoli

Instructions

* Use salt, pepper, and olive oil to season the chicken breasts.
* In a pan over medium heat, warm the olive oil. When the chicken breasts are golden brown on both sides, add them and simmer.
* Take out the chicken and place it aside from the pan.
* In the same pan, sauté the onion and garlic for two to three minutes, or until softened.
* Add the yogurt, turmeric powder, lemon juice, and chicken broth.After whisking everything together, simmer.
* Simmer the sauce for five minutes, stirring now and again.
* Fill the pan with the cooked chicken and broccoli florets.Put the pot back on to simmer and cook for an additional five minutes, or until the chicken is cooked through and the broccoli is soft.
* Place the cooked quinoa on top of the chicken and broccoli...

Nutritional Value:

- Calories: 400
- Fiber: 7 grams
- Protein: 30 grams
- Fat: 15 grams (healthy fats from yogurt and olive oil)
- Anti-inflammatory benefits: Turmeric, lemon, broccoli
- Protein and nutrients: Quinoa and chicken

Spiced Lentil and Sweet Potato Soup with Whole-Wheat Bread

- **Prep Time:** 30 minutes
- **Serves:** 4

Ingredients

- 1 tsp olive oil
- 1/2 cup finely chopped onion; 2 minced garlic cloves
- one cup of washed green lentils
- One chopped and peeled sweet potato and four cups of vegetable broth

- One teaspoon of cumin powder
- half a teaspoon of coriander powder
- One-fourth teaspoon of chili powder
- To taste, add salt and pepper.
- Whole wheat crackers to dip in

Instructions

- In a pot over medium heat, warm the olive oil. Add the onion and garlic, and simmer for about 5 minutes, or until softened.
- Include the lentils, broth, chili powder, sweet potato, cumin, and coriander along with salt and pepper. Once the lentils and sweet potato are soft, bring to a boil, lower the heat, and simmer for 20 to 25 minutes.
- For a thicker consistency, use an immersion blender or blender to purée half of the soup.
- Provide warm, dipping servings with whole-wheat bread.

Nutritional Value:

- Calories: 250 per serving
- Fiber: 8 grams per serving
- Protein: 15 grams per serving

- Iron and folate: Rich in lentils
- Vitamin A and beta-carotene: From sweet potato
- Spices contain antioxidants.

- Extra Tips: Feel free to alter these recipes to suit your dietary requirements and preferences.
- Utilize your leftovers! For a week's worth of lunches, roast additional veggies for your Thai curry or prepare a double pot of lentil soup.
- Remember to stay hydrated! Water consumption is crucial for healthy digestion and general wellbeing.

Chapter 7: Snacks and Desserts Recipes

No-Bake Energy Bites with Berries and Nuts

- **Prep Time:** 10 minutes
- **Makes:** 10-12 bites

Ingredients

- 1/2 cup of rolled oats
- One-fourth cup of almond, cashew, or peanut butter
- 1/4 cup maple syrup or honey
- One-fourth cup chia seeds
- 1/4 cup of chopped dried fruit, such as apricots, dates, or cranberries
- 1/4 cup of chopped nuts, such as pecans, walnuts, or almonds

Instructions

- In a bowl, combine all the ingredient and well mix.

- Transfer the mixture to a baking sheet by rolling it into balls.
- Let cool for a minimum of half an hour prior to consumption.

Nutritional Value:
- Calories: 150 per bite
- Fiber: 4 grams per bite
- Protein: 4 grams per bite
- Fat: 8 grams per bite (healthy fats from nuts and nut butter)
- Antioxidants: From berries and nuts

Creamy Mango Chia Pudding with Coconut Milk

- **Prep Time:** 10 minutes (plus overnight soaking)
- **Serves:** 1

Ingredients
- One-fourth cup of chia seeds
- One cup of coconut milk without sugar
- 1/2 cup of frozen or fresh mango chopped

- One-fourth teaspoon of vanilla essence
- Taste-tested honey or maple syrup (optional)

Instructions
- In a jar or bowl, mix together chia seeds, coconut milk, mango, and vanilla extract. Stir well, cover, and refrigerate overnight.
- If preferred, top with more diced mango or another fruit in the morning. Optionally drizzle with maple syrup or honey.

Nutritional Value:
- Calories: 250
- Fiber: 10 grams
- Protein: 5 grams
- Fat: 15 grams (healthy fats from coconut milk)
- Vitamins and minerals: Packed with fruits and chia seeds

Baked Apple Slices with Cinnamon and Walnuts

- **Prep Time:** 15 minutes (plus baking time)

- **Serves:** 2

Ingredients
- 2 cored and thinly sliced apples
- 1/4 tsp ground cinnamon
- One tablespoon of finely chopped walnuts
- Half a teaspoon of maple syrup or honey (optional)

Instructions
- Set oven temperature to 175°C/350°F.
- Put apple slices in a baking sheet arrangement. Sprinkle with cinnamon and walnuts.
- Optionally drizzle with maple syrup or honey.
- Bake the apples for 15 to 20 minutes, or until they are soft and beginning to turn golden brown.

Nutritional Value:
- Calories: 150 per serving
- Fiber: 4 grams per serving
- Vitamin C and potassium: Rich in apples

- Antioxidants: From cinnamon and walnuts

Yogurt Parfait with Berries and Granola

- **Prep Time:** 5 minutes
- **Serves:** 1

Ingredients

- One cup of plain Greek yogurt, either lactose-free or low-fat
- 1/2 cup of mixed berries, either frozen or fresh
- 1/4 cup granola, if necessary made without gluten
- One-fourth teaspoon ground flaxseed, if desired

Instructions

- Arrange yogurt, granola, and berries in a parfait glass or bowl.
- Garnish with optional flaxseed and savor!

Nutritional Value:

- Calories: 250
- Fiber: 5 grams
- Protein: 15 grams
- Fat: 10 grams (healthy fats from yogurt and granola)
- Probiotics: From yogurt

Dark Chocolate and Cherry Trail Mix

- **Prep Time:** 5 minutes
- **Makes:** 1-2 servings

Ingredients

- 1/4 cup dark chocolate chips (containing 70% or more cacao)
- one-fourth cup of dried cherries
- one-fourth cup almonds
- one-fourth cup of pumpkin seeds
- 1/4 cup of shredded coconut without sugar (optional)

Instructions

- In a bowl, combine all the ingredients and well mix.
- For up to a week, keep at room temperature in an airtight container.

Nutritional Value:

- Calories: 200 per serving
- Fiber: 2 grams per serving
- Protein: 4 grams per serving
- Fat: 12 grams per serving (healthy fats from dark chocolate and nuts)
- Antioxidants: From dark chocolate, cherries, and nuts

Additional Tips:

- Feel free to alter these recipes to suit your dietary requirements and preferences.
- Experiment with different fruits, nuts, and seeds in your snacks and sweets.
- Use natural sweeteners sparingly, such as honey or maple syrup.

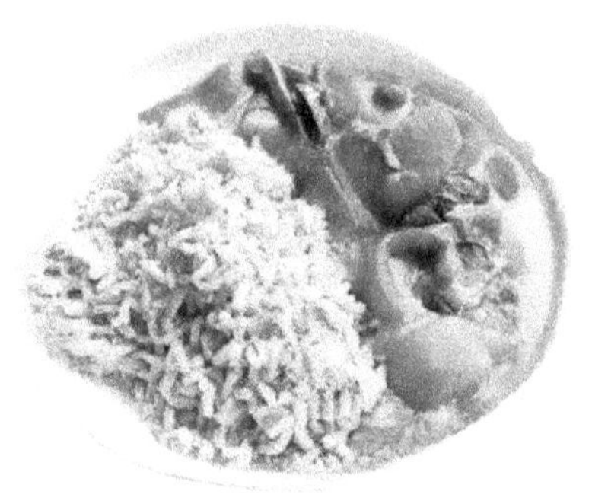

THAI VEGETABLE CURRY WITH BROWN RICE

Chapter 8: Smoothies

Green Powerhouse Smoothie

- **Prep Time:** 5 minutes
- **Serves:** 1

Ingredients
- 1 cup unsweetened almond milk, or any other preferred milk
- One handful of kale or spinach
- Half a ripe avocado
- half a banana
- 1/4 cup of chunks of frozen pineapple
- One tablespoon of optional collagen powder
- half a teaspoon of ginger powder
- A dash of turmeric

Instructions
- Put all the Ingredients in a blender and process until everything is creamy and smooth.
- Savor right now!

Nutritional Value:

- Calories: 300
- Fiber: 5 grams
- Protein: 10 grams (with collagen powder)
- Fat: 15 grams (healthy fats from avocado and almond milk)
- Antioxidants: From green leafy vegetables, pineapple, and turmeric
- Vitamins and minerals: Packed with avocado, banana, and leafy greens

Berrylicious Immunity Booster

- **Prep Time:** 5 minutes
- **Serves:** 1

Ingredients

- 1 cup low-fat or lactose-free plain Greek yogurt
- 1/2 cup of mixed berries, either frozen or fresh
- one-fourth cup blueberries
- 1/4 cup of cucumbers, chopped
- 1/4 cup of basic kefir, if desired

- One-fourth teaspoon of chia seeds
- A dash of cinnamon

Instructions
- Put all the Ingredients in a blender and process until everything is creamy and smooth.
- Top with fresh berries and chia seeds (optional).
- Have fun!

Nutritional Value:
- Calories: 250
- Fiber: 4 grams
- Protein: 20 grams (with kefir)
- Fat: 5 grams
- Probiotics: From yogurt and kefir (optional)
- Vitamin C and antioxidants: Rich in berries
- Anti-inflammatory benefits: Cinnamon

Tropical Detox Delight

- **Prep Time:** 5 minutes
- **Serves:** 1

Ingredients

- 1/2 mango, diced and peeled
- 1 cup unsweetened coconut water
- 1/4 cup pieces of pineapple
- 1/4 cup pieces of papaya
- 1/4 cup of cantaloupe, chopped
- One tablespoon of lime juice
- 1/4 cup of raw kale or spinach (optional)
- A pinch of ginger powder

Instructions

- Put all the Ingredients in a blender and process until everything is creamy and smooth.
- For an added nutritional boost, add optional spinach or kale.
- Have fun!

Nutritional Value:

- Calories: 200
- Fiber: 3 grams
- Vitamin C and A: Rich in tropical fruits

- Antioxidants: From pineapple, mango, and cantaloupe
- Electrolytes: Replenished by coconut water
- Digestive enzymes: From papaya

Creamy Pumpkin Spice Latte Smoothie

- **Prep Time:** 5 minutes
- **Serves:** 1

Ingredients
- 1 cup hot unsweetened almond milk
- Half a cup of boiled pumpkin puree
- 1/4 cup plain or vanilla Greek yogurt
- One-fourth teaspoon of pumpkin spice
- One-fourth teaspoon of vanilla essence
- A dash of cinnamon
- Taste-tested honey or maple syrup (optional)

Instructions
- Put all the Ingredients in a blender and process until everything is creamy and smooth.

- If preferred, drizzle with maple syrup or honey.
- Savor warm or cold!

Nutritional Value:
- Calories: 250
- Fiber: 3 grams
- Protein: 10 grams
- Vitamin A and E: Rich in pumpkin
- Antioxidants: From spices and pumpkin
- Probiotics: From yogurt (optional)

Chocolate Cherry Antioxidant Explosion

- **Prep Time:** 5 minutes
- **Serves:** 1

Ingredients
- 1 cup low-fat or lactose-free plain Greek yogurt
- half a cup of frozen cherries
- 1/4 cup chocolate powder, unsweetened
- one-fourth cup almond milk

- One-fourth teaspoon of extract from almonds
- A dash of sea salt

Instructions

- Put all the Ingredients in a blender and process until everything is creamy and smooth.
- For a thicker and colder consistency, add a few ice cubes (optional).
- For an added treat, top with chopped almonds or dark chocolate chips (optional).
- Savor this rich yet wholesome dessert!

Nutritional Value:

- Calories: 250
- Fiber: 4 grams
- Protein: 20 grams
- Fat: 5 grams
- Antioxidants: Rich in cherries and dark chocolate
- Probiotics: From yogurt
- Mood-boosting: From cocoa powder

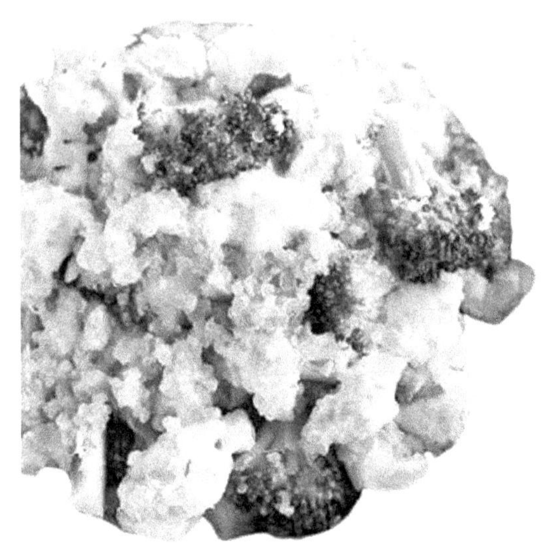

CREAMY LEMON CHICKEN WITH BROCCOLI AND QUINOA

Bonus Chapter: Portion control for optimal health and flare management

One of the most effective tools in your lupus diet toolbox is learning portion control. It involves more than just tracking calories; it also entails being aware of your body's demands, paying attention to your fullness signals, and choosing your meals carefully. Mindful portion control has a direct impact on your health and well-being when it comes to managing lupus by:

1. Reducing Inflammation: Overeating, especially refined carbs and processed meals, can promote inflammation in the body. You may naturally reduce your intake of these inflammatory triggers by regulating your portions, which can relax your body and possibly lower your chance of flare-ups.

2. Assisting with Weight Management: Since lupus drugs may cause weight gain, weight management is a crucial issue. Portion control eases joint pain, boosts vitality, and may even affect the efficacy of medications by assisting you in reaching and maintaining a healthy weight.

3. Improving Digestive Health: Eating too much can strain your digestive tract, causing pain and irritation. Meals that are smaller and better balanced facilitate digestion, which lessens discomfort and promotes gut health in general—a condition that is essential for optimum immunological performance.

4. Increasing Energy: Consuming a lot of food frequently causes blood sugar to rise and fall, which makes you tired and makes it harder to go about your everyday business. Regular, smaller meals that are balanced in terms of protein, fiber, and healthy fats give you long-lasting energy that keeps you moving and involved all day.

5. Encouraging Emotional Well-Being: Portion control and mindful eating techniques can support a healthy relationship with food and lessen tension and anxiety at mealtimes. This encourages mental health and gives you the ability to choose what and how much you consume with awareness.

Gaining Control Over Portion Size:

1. Accept Visual Cues: To naturally control your portion sizes, use smaller bowls and plates. Instead of using big serving dishes that encourage overfilling, place food directly onto plates.

2. Listen to Your Body: Be aware of your body's signals of hunger and fullness. Before grabbing for more, take your time eating and enjoy every taste, letting your body send out indications of fullness.

3. Arrange Your Meals: Making a meal and snack plan ahead of time helps you avoid impulsive eating and guarantees that you always have wholesome options on hand. Plan your snack portions in advance to prevent mindless snacking.

4. Read food labels carefully. Take note of serving sizes and calorie counts. This knowledge empowers you to choose portion sizes wisely, particularly when it comes to packaged goods.

5. Put Quality First: Give nutrient-dense natural foods the upper hand over processed ones. Naturally filling and low in calories, these meals support satiety and general well-being.

6. Embrace Variety: Even if the general norm may be to eat less quantities, make sure you obtain a range of nutrients. Your daily diet should contain a variety of fruits, vegetables, whole grains, lean meats, and healthy fats.

7. Eat Every Meal: Missing a meal can cause overindulgence in the future. Moderately sized meals and snacks on a regular basis help to stabilize your blood sugar levels and maintain a healthy metabolism.

8. Remain Hydrated: Throughout the day, sipping water can help reduce cravings and deceptive hunger sensations. Prioritize drinking water before grabbing food since often thirst might be confused for appetite.

9. Mindful Cooking: You frequently have better control over portion sizes when you cook at home.

Make use of smaller measuring spoons and cups, choose nutrient-preserving cooking techniques, and refrain from using too much oil or bad fats.

10. Celebrate Your Progress: Pay attention to the progress you're making in portion control and mindful eating. Honor minor accomplishments and don't let mistakes deter you from your goals. Long-term success requires self-compassion and persistence.

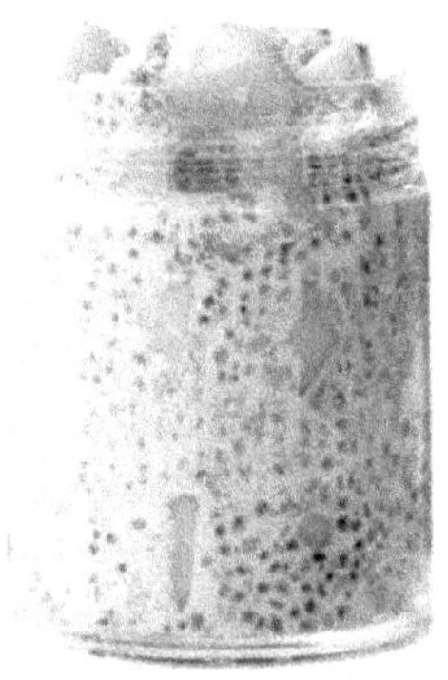

CREAMY MANGO CHIA PUDDING WITH COCONUT MILK

Conclusion

It is my aim that you would be motivated and equipped to create a wholesome and tasty Lupus Diet symphony in your own kitchen. Recall that every deliberate decision you make on your plate adds a harmonizing note to your well-being, which is a lovely composition.

Remember that food has the potential to heal, energize, and offer joy—whether you've experienced the warmth of creamy pumpkin spice lattes, the colorful dance of veggies in our Thai curry, or the soothing sweetness of dark chocolate and cherry delights.

This cookbook is simply the beginning of your culinary journey. Continue learning, experimenting, and creating your own unique blend of nutrients, flavors, and textures. Savor the distinct tune of your body, move in sync with the changing seasons, and rejoice in the harmonious blend of health that emerges from every thoughtful mouthful.

From the bottom of my dietitian's heart, I appreciate you joining me on this food journey. I am grateful for every page flipped, recipe tried, and mouthwatering moment enjoyed. Your commitment to your health inspires me to develop new tools and support people as they embark on their lupus diet adventures.

You Too Can Help

One of the most priceless gifts you could give me is your views and experiences. Every evaluation, communication, and culinary partnership is noted in the upcoming Lupus Diet Cookbook materials. Your voice helps me hone and develop future work, whether it's a soft symphony of gratitude or a bright blast of constructive criticism.

Therefore, if this cookbook touched you, please think about telling others about your experience. In addition to assisting others in discovering this oasis of delectable and nutritious dishes, your ratings give me essential information that help me create even more useful resources in the future.

One tasty mouthful at a time, let's continue creating the lovely symphony of wellbeing together.

With best wishes and eagerness for food,

**MILDRED A. KELLY
(AUTHOR LUPUS DIET COOKBOOK)**